Healing Soap Recipes
30 Homemade Soaps That Cure Skin Problems

Table of content

Introduction

You know germs are everywhere, and you know in order to stay healthy, you are going to have to keep clean. But, it seems that there is always something going on with your skin that drives you insane – whether you are dealing with burns, scraps, dry skin, irritation, or rashes.

The soaps on the market can be harsh on these conditions, making it harder for you to heal. But, you can't give up on using these soaps, or you are going to risk infections, illness, and a host of other problems.

So what are you going to do?

Clearly, the answer is to make your own soap.

But, you wonder, how are you going to do this – isn't soap difficult to make? Aren't there all kinds of harmful ingredients involved? Is there any way you can do it and not risk exposure to harmful chemicals?

If you have ever had any of these concerns, you have come to the right place. This book is going to show you everything you need to know to make your own soaps, regardless of what your skin irritation is.

Discover a host of different recipes, and create the soap that is going to get you back on track, and fall in love with being clean.

Chapter 1 – Healing Soaps for Dry Skin

Whether it is the cold of winter or the heat of summer, it seems that you can't get away from the dry skin that plagues you. Thankfully, you do have relief in sight, and with these soaps, you are going to get that moisture your dry skin so desperately needs.

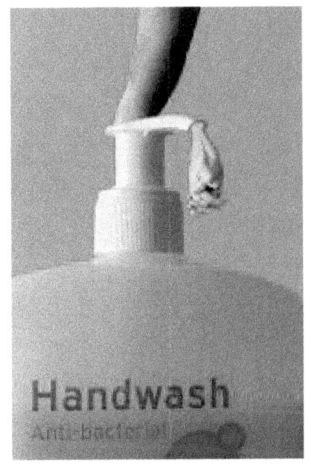

Moisture Extreme
What you will need:

12 drops chamomile essential oil

12 drops myrrh essential oil

1 tablespoon honey

1 cup unscented castile soap

2 tablespoons shea butter

1 tablespoon glycerin

¼ cup distilled water

Directions:

Using either a double boiler or a homemade double boiler, melt the shea butter until it is completely smooth. Add in the remaining ingredients (except for the essential oils) one at a time, mixing them in thoroughly (you don't want there to be any lumps in the mix at all.)

After you have thoroughly blended the ingredients, add the essential oils in next, and also stir them in until the mix is completely smooth. Remove from heat and allow to cool slightly, stirring the entire time.

Once the soap has cooled enough to touch, transfer from your double boiler to a soap dispenser, and use frequently on any dry skin you have.

Soothing Oasis
What you will need:

10 drops sunflower essential oil

10 drops sandalwood oil

1 tablespoon honey

1 cup unscented castile soap

2 tablespoons shea butter

1 tablespoon glycerin

¼ cup distilled water

Directions:

Using either a double boiler or a homemade double boiler, melt the shea butter until it is completely smooth. Add in the remaining ingredients (except for the essential oils) one at a time, mixing them in thoroughly (you don't want there to be any lumps in the mix at all.)

After you have thoroughly blended the ingredients, add the essential oils in next, and also stir them in until the mix is completely smooth. Remove from heat and allow to cool slightly, stirring the entire time.

Once the soap has cooled enough to touch, transfer from your double boiler to a soap dispenser, and use frequently on any dry skin you have.

Skip to My Loo
What you will need:

10 drops juniper berry essential oil

12 drops clove oil

1 tablespoon honey

1 cup unscented castile soap

2 tablespoons shea butter

1 tablespoon glycerin

¼ cup distilled water

Directions:

Using either a double boiler or a homemade double boiler, melt the shea butter until it is completely smooth. Add in the remaining ingredients (except for the essential oils) one at a time, mixing them in thoroughly (you don't want there to be any lumps in the mix at all.)

After you have thoroughly blended the ingredients, add the essential oils in next, and also stir them in until the mix is completely smooth. Remove from heat and allow to cool slightly, stirring the entire time.

Once the soap has cooled enough to touch, transfer from your double boiler to a soap dispenser, and use frequently on any dry skin you have.

Silken Fingers
What you will need:

18 drops vanilla essential oil

12 drops lavender essential oil

1 tablespoon honey

1 cup unscented castile soap

2 tablespoons shea butter

1 tablespoon glycerin

¼ cup distilled water

Directions:

Using either a double boiler or a homemade double boiler, melt the shea butter until it is completely smooth. Add in the remaining ingredients (except for the essential oils) one at a time, mixing them in thoroughly (you don't want there to be any lumps in the mix at all.)

After you have thoroughly blended the ingredients, add the essential oils in next, and also stir them in until the mix is completely smooth. Remove from heat and allow to cool slightly, stirring the entire time.

Once the soap has cooled enough to touch, transfer from your double boiler to a soap dispenser, and use frequently on any dry skin you have.

Happy Hands
What you will need:

10 drops rose essential oil

10 drops myrrh essential oil

1 tablespoon honey

1 cup unscented castile soap

2 tablespoons shea butter

1 tablespoon glycerin

¼ cup distilled water

Directions:

Using either a double boiler or a homemade double boiler, melt the shea butter until it is completely smooth. Add in the remaining ingredients (except for the essential oils) one at a time, mixing them in thoroughly (you don't want there to be any lumps in the mix at all.)

After you have thoroughly blended the ingredients, add the essential oils in next, and also stir them in until the mix is completely smooth. Remove from heat and allow to cool slightly, stirring the entire time.

Once the soap has cooled enough to touch, transfer from your double boiler to a soap dispenser, and use frequently on any dry skin you have.

Better than Oil

What you will need:

12 drops grapefruit oil

10 drops sunflower essential oil

1 tablespoon honey

1 cup unscented castile soap

2 tablespoons shea butter

1 tablespoon glycerin

¼ cup distilled water

Directions:

Using either a double boiler or a homemade double boiler, melt the shea butter until it is completely smooth. Add in the remaining ingredients (except for the essential oils) one at a time, mixing them in thoroughly (you don't want there to be any lumps in the mix at all.)

After you have thoroughly blended the ingredients, add the essential oils in next, and also stir them in until the mix is completely smooth. Remove from heat and allow to cool slightly, stirring the entire time.

Once the soap has cooled enough to touch, transfer from your double boiler to a soap dispenser, and use frequently on any dry skin you have.

Chapter 2 – Healing Soaps for Cuts, Scrapes, and Scratches

Whether it's you or your kids, there always seems to be someone with a scrape or a scratch in the house. With this soap, you can rest assured that those little injuries will heal quickly, ensuring you get a speedy recovery.

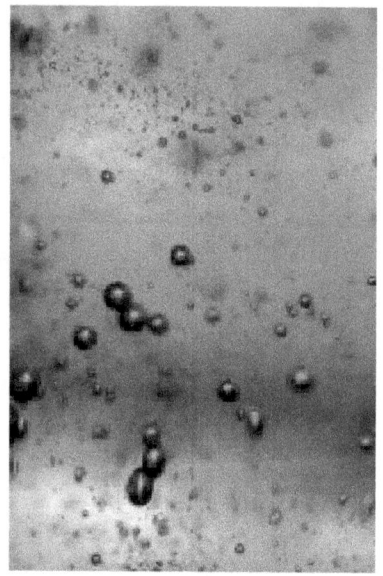

Clean Freak
What you will need:

12 drops cinnamon oil

6 drops orange oil

¼ teaspoon tea tree oil

1 cup unscented castile soap

1 tablespoon glycerin

¼ cup distilled water

Directions:

Using either a double boiler or a homemade double boiler, combine all ingredients (except for the essential oils) one at a time, mixing them together thoroughly.

After you have thoroughly blended the ingredients, add the essential oils in next, and also stir them in until the mix is completely smooth. Remove from heat and allow to cool slightly, stirring the entire time.

Once the soap has cooled enough to touch, transfer from your double boiler to a soap dispenser, and use frequently on any cuts or scrapes you have.

Kiss it Better
What you will need:

10 drops ylang ylang oil

12 drops cedar oil

¼ teaspoon tea tree oil

1 cup unscented castile soap

1 tablespoon glycerin

¼ cup distilled water

Directions:

Using either a double boiler or a homemade double boiler, combine all ingredients (except for the essential oils) one at a time, mixing them together thoroughly.

After you have thoroughly blended the ingredients, add the essential oils in next, and also stir them in until the mix is completely smooth. Remove from heat and allow to cool slightly, stirring the entire time.

Once the soap has cooled enough to touch, transfer from your double boiler to a soap dispenser, and use frequently on any cuts or scrapes you have.

Speed Healer
What you will need:

10 drops sage oil

10 drops clary sage oil

¼ teaspoon tea tree oil

1 cup unscented castile soap

1 tablespoon glycerin

¼ cup distilled water

Directions:

Using either a double boiler or a homemade double boiler, combine all ingredients (except for the essential oils) one at a time, mixing them together thoroughly.

After you have thoroughly blended the ingredients, add the essential oils in next, and also stir them in until the mix is completely smooth. Remove from heat and allow to cool slightly, stirring the entire time.

Once the soap has cooled enough to touch, transfer from your double boiler to a soap dispenser, and use frequently on any cuts or scrapes you have.

The Perfect Touch

What you will need:

12 drops lavender oil

10 drops sandalwood oil

¼ teaspoon tea tree oil

1 cup unscented castile soap

1 tablespoon glycerin

¼ cup distilled water

Directions:

Using either a double boiler or a homemade double boiler, combine all ingredients (except for the essential oils) one at a time, mixing them together thoroughly.

After you have thoroughly blended the ingredients, add the essential oils in next, and also stir them in until the mix is completely smooth. Remove from heat and allow to cool slightly, stirring the entire time.

Once the soap has cooled enough to touch, transfer from your double boiler to a soap dispenser, and use frequently on any cuts or scrapes you have.

Mother's Choice

What you will need:

10 drops lemongrass oil

10 drops lemon oil

¼ teaspoon tea tree oil

1 cup unscented castile soap

1 tablespoon glycerin

¼ cup distilled water

Directions:

Using either a double boiler or a homemade double boiler, combine all ingredients (except for the essential oils) one at a time, mixing them together thoroughly.

After you have thoroughly blended the ingredients, add the essential oils in next, and also stir them in until the mix is completely smooth. Remove from heat and allow to cool slightly, stirring the entire time.

Once the soap has cooled enough to touch, transfer from your double boiler to a soap dispenser, and use frequently on any cuts or scrapes you have.

Double Trouble

What you will need:

10 drops lemon oil

8 drops orange oil

¼ teaspoon tea tree oil

1 cup unscented castile soap

1 tablespoon glycerin

¼ cup distilled water

Directions:

Using either a double boiler or a homemade double boiler, combine all ingredients (except for the essential oils) one at a time, mixing them together thoroughly.

After you have thoroughly blended the ingredients, add the essential oils in next, and also stir them in until the mix is completely smooth. Remove from heat and allow to cool slightly, stirring the entire time.

Once the soap has cooled enough to touch, transfer from your double boiler to a soap dispenser, and use frequently on any cuts or scrapes you have.

Chapter 3 – Healing Soaps for Burns

No matter how careful you are in the kitchen, you are always risking being burned. When it does happen, you want relief, and you want it fast – and that's where these soaps come in. Wash your hands with these, and feel instant, soothing relief that will get you back in the game in no time.

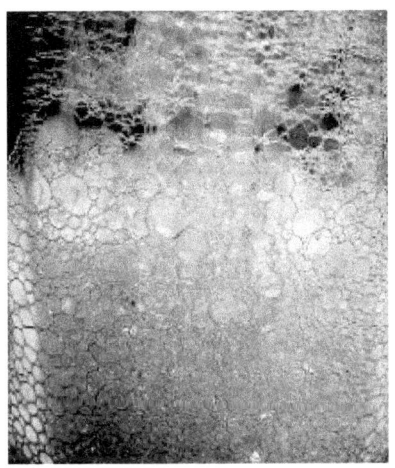

Baker's Best Friend
What you will need:

12 drops frankincense oil

10 drops jasmine oil

¼ cup aloe

1 tablespoon beeswax

1 cup unscented castile soap

1 tablespoon glycerin

¼ cup distilled water

Directions:

Using either a double boiler or a homemade double boiler, melt the beeswax until it is completely smooth. Add in the remaining ingredients (except for the essential oils) one at a time, mixing them in thoroughly (you don't want there to be any lumps in the mix at all.)

After you have thoroughly blended the ingredients, add the essential oils in next, and also stir them in until the mix is completely smooth. Remove from heat and allow to cool slightly, stirring the entire time.

Once the soap has cooled enough to touch, transfer from your double boiler to a soap dispenser, and use frequently on any burns you have.

The Fire Extinguisher
What you will need:

10 drops lavender oil

10 drops bergamot oil

¼ cup aloe

1 tablespoon beeswax

1 cup unscented castile soap

1 tablespoon glycerin

¼ cup distilled water

Directions:

Using either a double boiler or a homemade double boiler, melt the beeswax until it is completely smooth. Add in the remaining ingredients (except for the essential oils) one at a time, mixing them in thoroughly (you don't want there to be any lumps in the mix at all.)

After you have thoroughly blended the ingredients, add the essential oils in next, and also stir them in until the mix is completely smooth. Remove from heat and allow to cool slightly, stirring the entire time.

Once the soap has cooled enough to touch, transfer from your double boiler to a soap dispenser, and use frequently on any burns you have.

Burn Be Gone
What you will need:

12 drops tea tree oil

10 drops neem oil

¼ cup aloe

1 tablespoon beeswax

1 cup unscented castile soap

1 tablespoon glycerin

¼ cup distilled water

Directions:

Using either a double boiler or a homemade double boiler, melt the beeswax until it is completely smooth. Add in the remaining ingredients (except for the essential oils) one at a time, mixing them in thoroughly (you don't want there to be any lumps in the mix at all.)

After you have thoroughly blended the ingredients, add the essential oils in next, and also stir them in until the mix is completely smooth. Remove from heat and allow to cool slightly, stirring the entire time.

Once the soap has cooled enough to touch, transfer from your double boiler to a soap dispenser, and use frequently on any burns you have.

Splash
What you will need:

12 drops vetiver oil

10 drops sandalwood oil

¼ cup aloe

1 tablespoon beeswax

1 cup unscented castile soap

1 tablespoon glycerin

¼ cup distilled water

Directions:

Using either a double boiler or a homemade double boiler, melt the beeswax until it is completely smooth. Add in the remaining ingredients (except for the essential oils) one at a time, mixing them in thoroughly (you don't want there to be any lumps in the mix at all.)

After you have thoroughly blended the ingredients, add the essential oils in next, and also stir them in until the mix is completely smooth. Remove from heat and allow to cool slightly, stirring the entire time.

Once the soap has cooled enough to touch, transfer from your double boiler to a soap dispenser, and use frequently on any burns you have.

Cooling Contact
What you will need:

12 drops peppermint oil

10 drops eucalyptus oil

¼ cup aloe

1 tablespoon beeswax

1 cup unscented castile soap

1 tablespoon glycerin

¼ cup distilled water

Directions:

Using either a double boiler or a homemade double boiler, melt the beeswax until it is completely smooth. Add in the remaining ingredients (except for the essential oils) one at a time, mixing them in thoroughly (you don't want there to be any lumps in the mix at all.)

After you have thoroughly blended the ingredients, add the essential oils in next, and also stir them in until the mix is completely smooth. Remove from heat and allow to cool slightly, stirring the entire time.

Once the soap has cooled enough to touch, transfer from your double boiler to a soap dispenser, and use frequently on any burns you have.

Miracle Cream
What you will need:

12 drops goldenseal oil

10 drops lemongrass oil

¼ cup aloe

1 tablespoon beeswax

1 cup unscented castile soap

1 tablespoon glycerin

¼ cup distilled water

Directions:

Using either a double boiler or a homemade double boiler, melt the beeswax until it is completely smooth. Add in the remaining ingredients (except for the essential oils) one at a time, mixing them in thoroughly (you don't want there to be any lumps in the mix at all.)

After you have thoroughly blended the ingredients, add the essential oils in next, and also stir them in until the mix is completely smooth. Remove from heat and allow to cool slightly, stirring the entire time.

Once the soap has cooled enough to touch, transfer from your double boiler to a soap dispenser, and use frequently on any burns you have.

Chapter 4 – Healing Soaps for Rashes

Rashes seem to come out of nowhere. They can be a result of an allergen, some sort of irritant, or even plants. When you have a rash of any kind, you want nothing more than to just get rid of it.

With these soaps, you are going to see your rashes disappear in no time at all, and be back to feeling like your good old self.

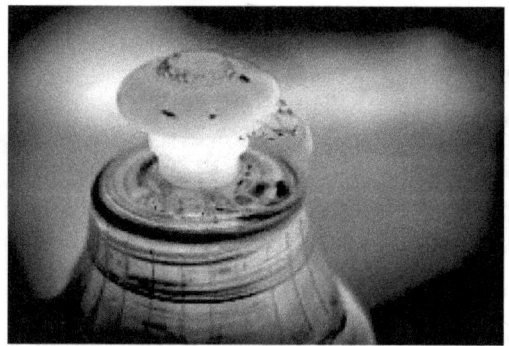

Spot Check

What you will need:

12 drops frankincense oil

10 drops myrrh oil

¼ cup aloe

1 tablespoon honey

1 tablespoon beeswax

1 cup unscented castile soap

1 tablespoon glycerin

¼ cup goat milk

Directions:

Using either a double boiler or a homemade double boiler, melt the beeswax until it is completely smooth. Add in the remaining ingredients (except for the essential oils) one at a time, mixing them in thoroughly (you don't want there to be any lumps in the mix at all.)

After you have thoroughly blended the ingredients, add the essential oils in next, and also stir them in until the mix is completely smooth. Remove from heat and allow to cool slightly, stirring the entire time.

Once the soap has cooled enough to touch, transfer from your double boiler to a soap dispenser, and use frequently on any rashes you have.

Rash Wash
What you will need:

12 drops chamomile oil

9 drops lavender oil

¼ cup aloe

1 tablespoon honey

1 tablespoon beeswax

1 cup unscented castile soap

1 tablespoon glycerin

¼ cup goat milk

Directions:

Using either a double boiler or a homemade double boiler, melt the beeswax until it is completely smooth. Add in the remaining ingredients (except for the essential oils) one at a time, mixing them in thoroughly (you don't want there to be any lumps in the mix at all.)

After you have thoroughly blended the ingredients, add the essential oils in next, and also stir them in until the mix is completely smooth. Remove from heat and allow to cool slightly, stirring the entire time.

Once the soap has cooled enough to touch, transfer from your double boiler to a soap dispenser, and use frequently on any rashes you have.

Itch It
What you will need:

12 drops peppermint oil

12 drops spearmint oil

¼ cup aloe

1 tablespoon honey

1 tablespoon beeswax

1 cup unscented castile soap

1 tablespoon glycerin

¼ cup goat milk

Directions:

Using either a double boiler or a homemade double boiler, melt the beeswax until it is completely smooth. Add in the remaining ingredients (except for the essential oils) one at a time, mixing them in thoroughly (you don't want there to be any lumps in the mix at all.)

After you have thoroughly blended the ingredients, add the essential oils in next, and also stir them in until the mix is completely smooth. Remove from heat and allow to cool slightly, stirring the entire time.

Once the soap has cooled enough to touch, transfer from your double boiler to a soap dispenser, and use frequently on any rashes you have.

Something Swell
What you will need:

10 drops geranium oil

10 drops ylang ylang oil

¼ cup aloe

1 tablespoon honey

1 tablespoon beeswax

1 cup unscented castile soap

1 tablespoon glycerin

¼ cup goat milk

Directions:

Using either a double boiler or a homemade double boiler, melt the beeswax until it is completely smooth. Add in the remaining ingredients (except for the essential oils) one at a time, mixing them in thoroughly (you don't want there to be any lumps in the mix at all.)

After you have thoroughly blended the ingredients, add the essential oils in next, and also stir them in until the mix is completely smooth. Remove from heat and allow to cool slightly, stirring the entire time.

Once the soap has cooled enough to touch, transfer from your double boiler to a soap dispenser, and use frequently on any rashes you have.

Happy Days
What you will need:

12 drops helychirsum oil

8 drops vetiver oil

¼ cup aloe

1 tablespoon honey

1 tablespoon beeswax

1 cup unscented castile soap

1 tablespoon glycerin

¼ cup goat milk

Directions:

Using either a double boiler or a homemade double boiler, melt the beeswax until it is completely smooth. Add in the remaining ingredients (except for the essential oils) one at a time, mixing them in thoroughly (you don't want there to be any lumps in the mix at all.)

After you have thoroughly blended the ingredients, add the essential oils in next, and also stir them in until the mix is completely smooth. Remove from heat and allow to cool slightly, stirring the entire time.

Once the soap has cooled enough to touch, transfer from your double boiler to a soap dispenser, and use frequently on any rashes you have.

Spring Fever

What you will need:

12 drops spearmint oil

12 drops wintergreen oil

¼ cup aloe

1 tablespoon honey

1 tablespoon beeswax

1 cup unscented castile soap

1 tablespoon glycerin

¼ cup goat milk

Directions:

Using either a double boiler or a homemade double boiler, melt the beeswax until it is completely smooth. Add in the remaining ingredients (except for the essential oils) one at a time, mixing them in thoroughly (you don't want there to be any lumps in the mix at all.)

After you have thoroughly blended the ingredients, add the essential oils in next, and also stir them in until the mix is completely smooth. Remove from heat and allow to cool slightly, stirring the entire time.

Once the soap has cooled enough to touch, transfer from your double boiler to a soap dispenser, and use frequently on any rashes you have.

Chapter 5 – Healing Soaps for Irritated Skin

Let's face it, there are times when you skin is irritated, and you just don't know why. Here are a few recipes for soothing oils that will leave your skin feeling back to its wonderful self.

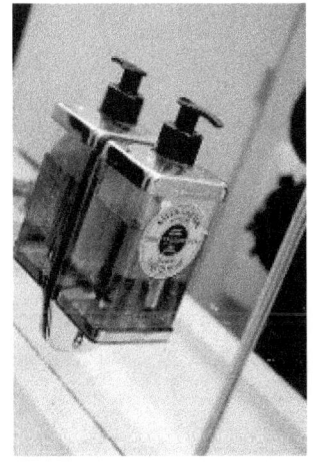

That Hits the Spot
What you will need:

12 drops eucalyptus oil

9 drops geranium oil

2 tablespoons olive oil

1 cup unscented castile soap

2 tablespoons shea butter

1 tablespoon glycerin

¼ cup distilled water

Directions:

Using either a double boiler or a homemade double boiler, melt the shea butter until it is completely smooth. Add in the remaining ingredients (except for the essential oils) one at a time, mixing them in thoroughly (you don't want there to be any lumps in the mix at all.)

After you have thoroughly blended the ingredients, add the essential oils in next, and also stir them in until the mix is completely smooth. Remove from heat and allow to cool slightly, stirring the entire time.

Once the soap has cooled enough to touch, transfer from your double boiler to a soap dispenser, and use frequently on any irritated skin you have.

Going Green
What you will need:

12 drops tea tree oil

10 drops sage oil

2 tablespoons olive oil

1 cup unscented castile soap

2 tablespoons shea butter

1 tablespoon glycerin

¼ cup distilled water

Directions:

Using either a double boiler or a homemade double boiler, melt the shea butter until it is completely smooth. Add in the remaining ingredients (except for the essential oils) one at a time, mixing them in thoroughly (you don't want there to be any lumps in the mix at all.)

After you have thoroughly blended the ingredients, add the essential oils in next, and also stir them in until the mix is completely smooth. Remove from heat and allow to cool slightly, stirring the entire time.

Once the soap has cooled enough to touch, transfer from your double boiler to a soap dispenser, and use frequently on any irritated skin you have.

The Adventurer's Tonic
What you will need:

12 drops chamomile oil

11 drops bergamot oil

2 tablespoons olive oil

1 cup unscented castile soap

2 tablespoons shea butter

1 tablespoon glycerin

¼ cup distilled water

Directions:

Using either a double boiler or a homemade double boiler, melt the shea butter until it is completely smooth. Add in the remaining ingredients (except for the essential oils) one at a time, mixing them in thoroughly (you don't want there to be any lumps in the mix at all.)

After you have thoroughly blended the ingredients, add the essential oils in next, and also stir them in until the mix is completely smooth. Remove from heat and allow to cool slightly, stirring the entire time.

Once the soap has cooled enough to touch, transfer from your double boiler to a soap dispenser, and use frequently on any irritated skin you have.

Miraculous Magic
What you will need:

8 drops neem oil

12 drops vetiver oil

2 tablespoons olive oil

1 cup unscented castile soap

2 tablespoons shea butter

1 tablespoon glycerin

¼ cup distilled water

Directions:

Using either a double boiler or a homemade double boiler, melt the shea butter until it is completely smooth. Add in the remaining ingredients (except for the essential oils) one at a time, mixing them in thoroughly (you don't want there to be any lumps in the mix at all.)

After you have thoroughly blended the ingredients, add the essential oils in next, and also stir them in until the mix is completely smooth. Remove from heat and allow to cool slightly, stirring the entire time.

Once the soap has cooled enough to touch, transfer from your double boiler to a soap dispenser, and use frequently on any irritated skin you have.

Wash It Off
What you will need:

12 drops lavender oil

8 drops rose oil

2 tablespoons olive oil

1 cup unscented castile soap

2 tablespoons shea butter

1 tablespoon glycerin

¼ cup distilled water

Directions:

Using either a double boiler or a homemade double boiler, melt the shea butter until it is completely smooth. Add in the remaining ingredients (except for the essential oils) one at a time, mixing them in thoroughly (you don't want there to be any lumps in the mix at all.)

After you have thoroughly blended the ingredients, add the essential oils in next, and also stir them in until the mix is completely smooth. Remove from heat and allow to cool slightly, stirring the entire time.

Once the soap has cooled enough to touch, transfer from your double boiler to a soap dispenser, and use frequently on any irritated skin you have.

The Soothing Slime
What you will need:

12 drops rose oil

10 drops rosewood oil

2 tablespoons olive oil

1 cup unscented castile soap

2 tablespoons shea butter

1 tablespoon glycerin

¼ cup distilled water

Directions:

Using either a double boiler or a homemade double boiler, melt the shea butter until it is completely smooth. Add in the remaining ingredients (except for the essential oils) one at a time, mixing them in thoroughly (you don't want there to be any lumps in the mix at all.)

After you have thoroughly blended the ingredients, add the essential oils in next, and also stir them in until the mix is completely smooth. Remove from heat and allow to cool slightly, stirring the entire time.

Once the soap has cooled enough to touch, transfer from your double boiler to a soap dispenser, and use frequently on any irritated skin you have.

Conclusion

There you have it, everything you need to make your own soaps and treat any kind of skin condition you may experience. I hope this book gives you the inspiration that you need to make your own soaps, no matter what your skin condition is.

This book has everything you need to take care of all your skin care ailments, and it's going to change the way you view the soap that you make. Get ready to pamper yourself in a whole new way.

Good luck, and have a happy cleaning!

FREE Bonus Reminder

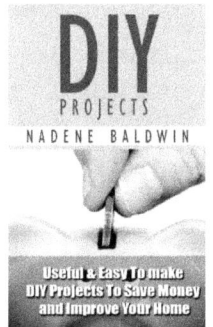

If you have not grabbed it yet, please go ahead and download your special bonus report *"DIY Projects. 13 Useful & Easy To Make DIY Projects To Save Money & Improve Your Home!"*

Simply Click the Button Below

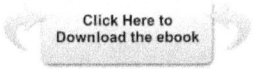

OR **Go to This Page**

http://diyhomecraft.com/free

BONUS #2: More Free & Discounted Books or Products

Do you want to receive more Free/Discounted Books or Products?

We have a mailing list where we send out our new Books or Products when they go free or with a discount on Amazon. Click on the link below to sign up for Free & Discount Book & Product Promotions.

=> Sign Up for Free & Discount Book & Product Promotions <=

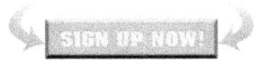

OR Go to this URL

http://zbit.ly/1WBb1Ek

www.ingramcontent.com/pod-product-compliance
Lightning Source LLC
Chambersburg PA
CBHW071145280526
45787CB00003B/1410